Surrogacy in the US

Your How-To Guide for Intended Parents on Navigating the Surrogacy Process, Costs, and More

Ian Unger

Contents

Introduction: About the Author

Starting a family is one of the most exciting and emotional journeys in life, and for me, it was no different. But when that path involves surrogacy—especially across borders—it can quickly become overwhelming, complex, and filled with uncertainties. I'm Ian, and I've navigated this journey myself. As an American living in Europe with my husband, Alex, who is from Spain, we faced the complexities of becoming parents through surrogacy in the United States. We experienced firsthand the questions, concerns, and challenges that can arise, but we also discovered ways to navigate them effectively.

Now, I want to share those insights with you. With this book, my goal is to provide the guidance and information you need to feel confident, prepared, and in control of your surrogacy journey—no matter where in the world you're starting from.

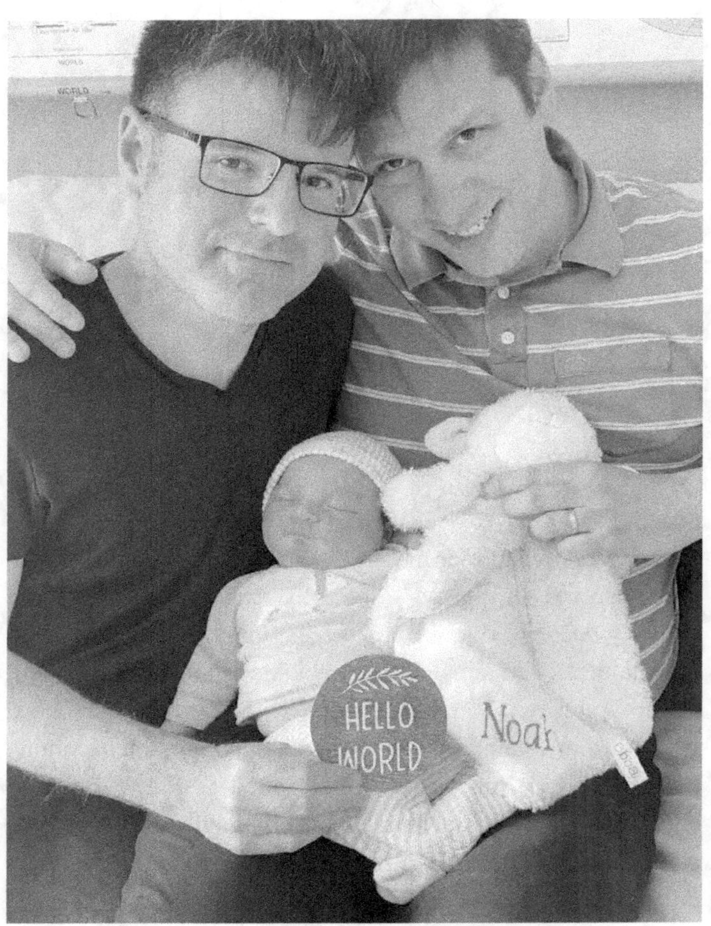

Our Story

My name is Ian, and my husband Alex and I are the proud parents of our amazing son, Noah, who was born via surrogacy in the United States. Originally from the US, I've lived in Europe since 2009, and Alex is from Spain. We navigated the complex journey of becoming parents across continents—a process that was both challenging and incredibly rewarding.

Every step of the way, we faced questions, uncertainties, and decisions that felt overwhelming, but our love for our future child kept us moving forward. I want to share that journey with you, along with the lessons we've learned, so that your path to parenthood can be smoother and more straight-forward.

Purpose of This Book

This book is designed to be your comprehensive guide through the surrogacy process, especially if you are considering surrogacy in the United States. Whether you're feeling uncertain about where to start or need clear answers to specific questions, this guide will offer the insights, tools, and strategies you need to feel empowered every step of the way. My goal is to arm you with the knowledge, tools, and strategies to make informed decisions, avoid common pitfalls, and feel more in control of your journey. Whether you're only now beginning to explore surrogacy or already deep into the planning stage, this guide is here to simplify the process, clarify what you need to know, and give you actionable steps to follow.

Why I Wrote This Book

Our journey through surrogacy taught us that the path to parenthood isn't always straightforward, and it's rarely a one-size-fits-all experience. From understanding legal complexities to managing costs, I realized there were so many ways to get sidetracked or overwhelmed. This book is my way of sharing the insights, lessons, and strategies we learned along the way so that others can embark on their journey with greater confidence and clarity. Throughout this book, you'll

find references to helpful resources from Surrogacy Guidance, a service I founded to support intended parents in navigating the surrogacy process. Our goal is to be with you every
step of the way, offering expert advice, resources, and a
supportive community to help make your surrogacy journey
as smooth as possible. For more information, visit www.surro
gacyguidance.com.

What This Book Will Offer You

This book serves as a comprehensive guide for intended
parents, particularly those considering surrogacy in the
United States. From understanding the costs and choosing the
right providers to managing legal requirements and cross-
border challenges, this book covers everything you need to
know to make informed decisions. My goal is to demystify
the process and provide practical advice to help you save
time, money, and stress. Here's what you'll learn:

- **Understanding the Surrogacy Process**: A step-by-
  step guide to navigating surrogacy in the United
  States, from initial research to bringing your baby
  home.
- **Cost-Saving Strategies**: Proven techniques to
  manage and reduce costs without compromising on
  quality or safety, ensuring your surrogacy journey is
  both affordable and effective.
- **Legal and Cross-Border Considerations**: What
  international intended parents need to know about
  legalities, insurance, and more.
- **Common Pitfalls & How to Avoid Them**: Real-
  world tips on how to sidestep common challenges in
  the surrogacy journey.

- **Building Your Surrogacy Support Network**: How to find the right team to support you, from agencies and clinics to legal professionals and counselors.

Who This Book is For

Whether you're just beginning to explore surrogacy or already deep into planning, this guide is designed to support all intended parents seeking reliable information and guidance. No matter your background, circumstances, or where you are in your journey, this book can be your trusted companion. It is especially beneficial for:

- Same-sex couples who want to build a family through surrogacy.
- Single parents embarking on the journey solo.
- Heterosexual couples facing infertility or other reproductive challenges.
- Both US-based and international intended parents navigating the complexities of cross-border surrogacy.

No matter your situation, this book will empower you with a clear understanding of surrogacy in the US, helping you take confident steps forward.

What You'll Gain

By the end of this book, you will have a detailed understanding of the surrogacy process in the United States, including financial, legal, and logistical aspects. You'll learn how to build a trusted team, avoid common pitfalls, and find cost-saving opportunities. Most importantly, you will gain the peace of mind that comes with knowing what to expect and how to prepare for this life-changing journey.

Conclusion

I encourage you to take your time reading through this book, revisiting sections as needed, and using the resources provided. Remember, the surrogacy journey may have its complexities, but with the right guidance, it can also be a beautiful and fulfilling experience. I invite you to visit Surrogacy Guidance for additional support, resources, and the opportunity to connect directly with experts who are ready to help you every step of the way.

Chapter 1
How to Understand Surrogacy

The surrogacy journey begins with a clear understanding of what it involves. Knowing the different types of surrogacy and their implications can help you make informed decisions that align with your needs, preferences, and legal requirements. This foundational knowledge will empower you to navigate the complexities ahead with confidence.

Surrogacy is an arrangement where a surrogate carries and births a child for another person or couple, known as the intended parents (IPs). There are four primary forms of surrogacy:

1.1 Gestational Surrogacy

Gestational surrogacy is the most common and widely accepted form of surrogacy today. In this arrangement, the surrogate becomes pregnant via in vitro fertilization (IVF), using the egg and sperm from the intended parents or donors. Because the egg is not from the surrogate, she has no genetic link to the child. This has become the standard in most countries due to its clear legal and emotional boundaries, making it easier to establish parentage for the intended parents.

For instance, in gestational surrogacy, a couple might use the mother's egg and the father's sperm, with the embryo implanted in the surrogate's womb. This arrangement ensures that the surrogate has no genetic connection to the child, which helps to avoid complications over parental rights.

The preference for gestational surrogacy stems from its legal clarity. Since the surrogate has no genetic link to the baby, it minimizes the risk of legal disputes over parental rights. This arrangement ensures that intended parents are recognized as the legal parents, which is especially important in states or countries with strict surrogacy laws.

1.2 Traditional Surrogacy

Traditional surrogacy is much less common and is legally and emotionally more complex. In this arrangement, the surrogate's own egg is fertilized with sperm from the intended father or donor, making her the genetic mother of the child. Due to the genetic link, traditional surrogacy can lead to legal disputes over parental rights, and it is less accepted in many places around the world. Because of these complications, traditional surrogacy has largely been replaced by gestational surrogacy.

In traditional surrogacy, the surrogate might use her own egg, making her the biological mother of the child. This genetic link can lead to emotional and legal complexities, which is why many intended parents and surrogacy professionals prefer gestational arrangements.

1.3 Altruistic Surrogacy

Altruistic surrogacy is when the surrogate agrees to carry a child for intended parents without financial compensation beyond medical expenses. This arrangement often stems from a personal connection or desire to help another family. While it may seem more straightforward, altruistic surrogacy still requires clear legal agreements to protect the rights of both the surrogate and intended parents.

1.4 Compensated Surrogacy

Compensated surrogacy involves the surrogate receiving financial compensation for her services, in addition to coverage for medical expenses. This is the most common form of surrogacy in many countries, as it provides the surrogate with fair compensation for her time, effort, and potential risks. Clear legal contracts are essential in compensated surrogacy to ensure that all parties understand their rights and responsibilities.

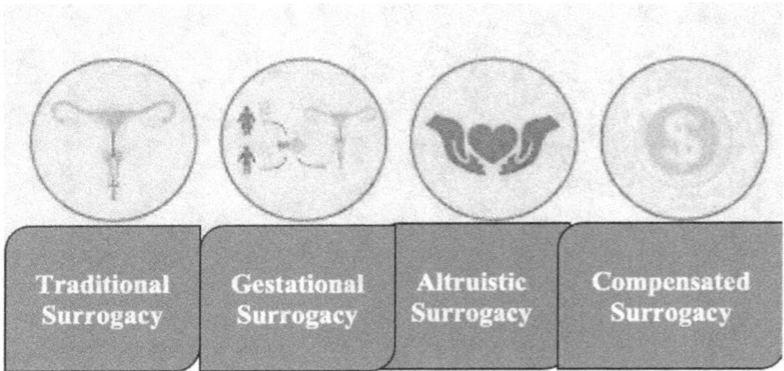

Now that you have a basic understanding of what surrogacy entails, the next step is to explore why the United States has emerged as the gold standard for surrogacy worldwide, and what makes it a preferred destination for intended parents from across the globe.

Chapter 2
Why the United States is the "Gold Standard" for Surrogacy

Choosing to grow your family through surrogacy is a life-changing decision, and for many intended parents around the world, the United States stands out as the preferred destination. But what makes the US the gold standard for surrogacy, especially when there are surrogacy programs in other countries that appear less expensive? The answer lies in a combination of legal, medical, and ethical factors that make the US the safest, most reliable, and well-regulated place to pursue surrogacy.

2.1 Legal Certainty and Protection for Intended Parents and Surrogates

One of the main reasons the US is a leading destination for surrogacy is the strong legal framework in place to protect both intended parents and surrogates. Unlike many countries where surrogacy may be illegal or operate in a legal grey area, several US states have established clear, enforceable laws that support surrogacy agreements.

- **Pre-Birth and Post-Birth Orders**: In states where surrogacy is well-regulated, intended parents can obtain pre-birth orders that establish their legal parentage before the child is born. This means the names of the intended parents go directly on the birth certificate, avoiding potential legal battles or complications after the child's birth. In other countries, this process can be much more complex, involving lengthy court procedures and unpredictable outcomes.

- **Surrogacy-Friendly States**: Not all US states are surrogacy-friendly, but those that are—such as California, Illinois, and Connecticut—have comprehensive laws that make the surrogacy process smooth and secure. These states allow compensated surrogacy and provide robust legal mechanisms to protect the rights of all parties involved, including ensuring that the surrogate understands her rights and responsibilities.

US Surrogacy Law by State

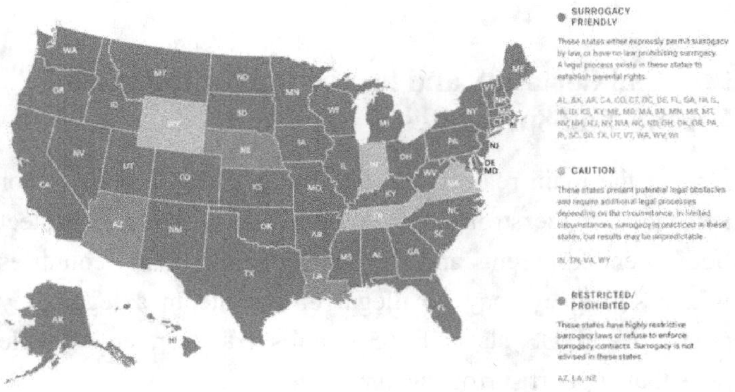

- **State Law Evolution**: Over the past decade, there has been a positive trend in the US where states have passed new laws to make surrogacy more accessible and legally secure. States like New York and New Jersey, which previously restricted surrogacy, have now enacted legislation that supports and regulates the practice. This shift has opened more legal paths for intended parents and solidified the US as a leader in surrogacy options.

- **Legal Protection for LGBTQ+ and Single Parents**: The US also leads in inclusivity, providing legal protection for LGBTQ+ couples and single intended parents. In many parts of the world, legal restrictions can prevent these individuals from pursuing surrogacy, but in the US, these protections are enshrined in law, offering a safe and welcoming environment for all types of families.

2.2 World-Class Medical Facilities and Expertise

Another key factor that makes the US the gold standard for surrogacy is the unparalleled quality of its medical facilities. The US has some of the most advanced fertility clinics in the world, with specialists who are highly experienced in assisted reproductive technology (ART), including in vitro fertilization (IVF) and embryo transfer.

- **Advanced Fertility Treatments**: US fertility clinics are often at the forefront of reproductive medicine, offering the latest advancements in fertility treatments, genetic screening, and embryo selection. This ensures a higher chance of success for intended parents, reducing the time, cost, and emotional strain of multiple cycles.

- **Strict Medical Regulations**: Medical practices in the US are regulated by authorities such as the Food and Drug Administration (FDA) and the Centers for Disease Control and Prevention (CDC). These regulations ensure high standards of care, ethical conduct, and the safety of both the surrogate and the child. Fertility clinics in the US must adhere to strict guidelines, providing peace of mind to intended parents who may not receive the same assurances elsewhere.

- **Access to Experienced Medical Professionals**: In addition to the facilities themselves, the US is home to some of the world's leading fertility specialists, embryologists, and surrogacy coordinators. The expertise available ensures that intended parents receive high-quality care throughout the surrogacy journey, from initial consultations to post-birth support.

2.3 Ethical Considerations and Surrogate Welfare

Ethical practices are a cornerstone of surrogacy in the US. The rights and well-being of surrogates are prioritized, with clear guidelines ensuring that they are treated fairly, ethically, and with respect. The process involves rigorous screening to ensure that surrogates are physically, emotionally, and financially prepared for the journey, which helps to protect all parties involved.

- **Informed Consent and Clear Agreements**: In the US, surrogates enter into the process voluntarily, with a comprehensive understanding of their rights and responsibilities. Contracts are thoroughly reviewed by legal professionals, and surrogates undergo psychological evaluations to ensure they are fully informed and committed. This focus on informed consent helps prevent exploitation and ensures that surrogates are genuinely motivated to help intended parents.

- **Comprehensive Screening**: Before a surrogacy agreement is finalized, potential surrogates go through extensive screening that includes:
  - **Medical Screening**: Surrogates must undergo thorough medical examinations to confirm they are in good health and capable of carrying a pregnancy safely. This ensures the surrogacy journey can proceed without unnecessary medical risks to both the surrogate and baby.
  - **Psychological Screening**: Psychological evaluations are conducted to assess the surrogate's mental and emotional readiness for the surrogacy process. This step helps confirm that the surrogate fully understands the emotional aspects of carrying a child for another family and is prepared to handle the complexities of the journey.
  - **Financial Screening**: Unlike in some countries, US surrogates must demonstrate financial stability before being accepted into the process. This requirement ensures that surrogacy is not a financial necessity but a voluntary, informed decision. While compensation is an essential component, it is not the primary motivator; surrogates are chosen for their desire to help

others build families, not because they are in financial distress.

- **Access to Healthcare and Compensation**: US surrogates are compensated not only for their time and effort but also receive comprehensive healthcare throughout the pregnancy. Compensation is regulated to ensure fairness, covering not just medical expenses but also lost wages, childcare, and other associated costs. This ensures surrogates are supported and that their own families do not face financial hardship as a result of their participation in the surrogacy process.

- **Commitment to Ethical Practices**: Fertility clinics, surrogacy agencies, and legal teams in the US are committed to ethical practices, adhering to established guidelines that prioritize the safety and welfare of all parties. This is in contrast to some countries where surrogacy may be less regulated, leading to ethical concerns and legal uncertainties. The emphasis on ethical standards ensures that intended parents and surrogates can proceed with confidence, knowing that they are supported by a framework designed to safeguard everyone's rights.

2.4 Experience, Mainstream Acceptance, and Accessibility

The United States has decades of experience with surrogacy, and this level of expertise translates into a smoother, more predictable process for intended parents. Over the years, surrogacy has become a widely accepted family-building option, and it is one of the few reproductive topics that, for the most part, remains apolitical in the US.

- **Experience and Expertise**: The US has been at the forefront of surrogacy for decades, meaning that clinics, agencies, and legal teams have honed their practices over many years. This experience reduces the risk of complications and increases the likelihood of a successful journey for intended parents.
- **Mainstream and Accepted**: Surrogacy is now a mainstream option in the US, discussed openly and without the stigma that might be found in other countries. While there are still some dark corners of the internet where the topic may be controversial, surrogacy is widely accepted across the US, making it a comfortable and supportive environment for intended parents.
- **Evolving and Improving State Laws**: Importantly, state laws in the US have been evolving over the past decade to make surrogacy more accessible, not less. States that once had restrictive or ambiguous surrogacy laws, like New York and Washington, have passed new legislation supporting the practice, reflecting a growing acceptance and support for diverse family structures. This continuous improvement in legal frameworks ensures that intended parents have more options and security than ever before.

2.5 Surrogacy-Friendly States: Well-Known and Under-the-Radar Options

Not all US states are surrogacy-friendly, but those that are—such as California, Illinois, and Connecticut—have comprehensive laws making the surrogacy process smooth and secure. These states allow compensated surrogacy and provide robust legal mechanisms to protect the rights of all parties involved, including ensuring that the surrogate understands her rights and responsibilities.

However, there are also several states that often fly under the radar but can offer more cost-effective options while still providing excellent support and legal frameworks for surrogacy. For intended parents looking for a balance of affordability and quality, consider these options:

- **Utah**: Where my son Noah was born, Utah has established a reliable and streamlined process for surrogacy, with clear legal protections for intended parents. Utah is also more affordable than some of the more well-known states, making it a great option for those seeking cost-effective solutions.
- **Texas**: Texas is a surrogacy-friendly state with well-defined laws that support compensated surrogacy agreements. It's also known for having high-quality medical facilities and a lower cost of living, which can reduce overall surrogacy expenses.
- **Florida**: Florida offers strong legal support for surrogacy, including pre-birth orders that secure the rights of intended parents before the child is born. With competitive clinic costs and an experienced network of professionals, it remains a popular choice.
- **Idaho**: Idaho has been a surrogacy hub for many years, known for its supportive legal environment and cost-effective surrogacy options. Recently, Idaho enhanced its appeal by becoming a pre-birth order state, allowing intended parents to secure their legal parentage before the child is born. This eliminates

the need for an adoption process, making Idaho a particularly attractive option for international intended parents who want to ensure a smooth and straightforward legal path. With its combination of affordability and a strong legal framework, Idaho remains a top choice for surrogacy.

These states, among others, offer strong legal frameworks, experienced medical facilities, and supportive environments for surrogacy, making them excellent alternatives for intended parents seeking more cost-effective options in the United States.

Conclusion

The United States is considered the gold standard for surrogacy because of its robust legal protections, world-class medical expertise, ethical standards, inclusivity, and extensive experience. While surrogacy can be an expensive and complex process, the peace of mind that comes with pursuing surrogacy in the US is unparalleled. Intended parents can trust that their rights will be protected, their surrogates will be treated with respect and care, and that they will have access to some of the best fertility care in the world.

For many, the US may seem like a costly option, but the benefits of legal certainty, medical excellence, and ethical practices far outweigh the initial expense. In the chapters ahead, we will explore more about the surrogacy process, costs, and ways to make this journey smoother and more affordable for all intended parents.

Chapter 3
Exploring Global Surrogacy Options: Costs, Risks, and Realities

When choosing a surrogacy program, cost is often a key consideration for many intended parents. However, it's crucial to remember that the safest and most secure options aren't always the cheapest. Understanding the hidden costs, risks, and legal realities across different countries can help you make an informed and responsible decision. This chapter provides an overview of surrogacy options across the globe and explains the hidden costs, risks, and challenges that can arise when pursuing surrogacy in other countries.

The following map illustrates the different regulations surrounding surrogacy in various European countries, highlighting where commercial surrogacy is allowed, where altruistic surrogacy is permitted, and where surrogacy is banned or not clearly regulated. Understanding these laws is crucial for intended parents when considering surrogacy options abroad.

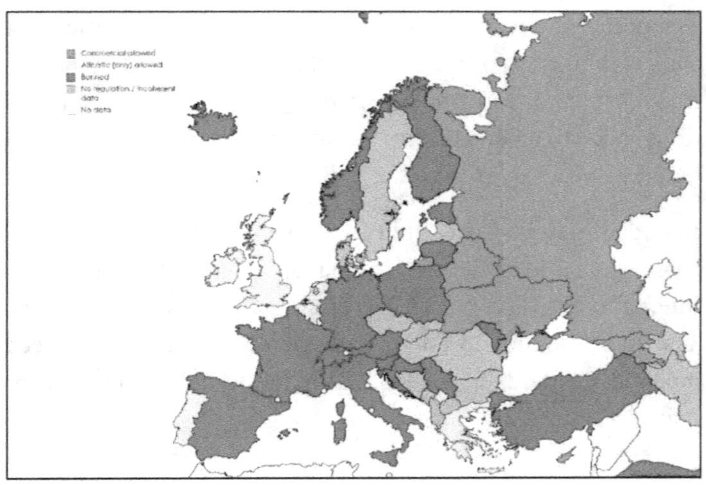

3.1 Overview of Surrogacy Options Around the World

Intended parents considering surrogacy have access to programs in various countries, each with its own set of regulations, legal frameworks, and price points. These countries can be grouped into several categories based on their legal, ethical, and operational structures:

3.2 United States: The Gold Standard

The United States is considered the gold standard for surrogacy. With robust legal protections, high-quality medical care, and inclusive practices, surrogacy in the US tends to be more expensive but offers a high degree of security and support. The United States offers clear legal protections that ensure intended parents' rights are safeguarded, high-quality medical care from world-class fertility clinics, and inclusive practices that accommodate a wide range of family structures. This combination of factors provides peace of mind and minimizes the chances of unexpected legal or medical complications, which is invaluable for many international intended parents.

Intended parents can find surrogacy-friendly states that cater to various needs, including legal recognition for international IPs, LGBTQ+ families, and single parents. The transparency, ethical considerations, and advanced medical standards make the US the preferred destination for many.

3.3 Western Countries with Altruistic Surrogacy Only

Some Western countries have legalized surrogacy but only allow it on an altruistic basis. This means that surrogates can only be reimbursed for expenses and are not compensated beyond that. This restriction often makes it difficult for intended parents to find a willing surrogate. Examples include:

- **Canada:** Surrogacy is legal, but only altruistic arrangements are permitted. While Canada has supportive legal frameworks, the restriction on compensation makes it challenging to find surrogates. The process can also be lengthy, adding to the overall complexity and uncertainty.
- **United Kingdom:** Similar to Canada, the UK only allows altruistic surrogacy. Surrogates can be reimbursed for reasonable expenses, but intended parents may find it difficult to locate a surrogate

willing to undergo the process without compensation. Legal parentage can also be complicated, requiring post-birth legal proceedings to transfer rights.

- **Australia, Sweden, and Denmark:** These countries also follow a similar model, allowing altruistic surrogacy but restricting any form of financial compensation. This can limit availability and make the surrogacy journey longer and less predictable.

3.4 Countries with Established Surrogacy Programs and Lower Costs

There are several countries where commercial surrogacy is legal, and the costs are significantly lower than in the United States. However, these countries often come with their own set of risks:

- **Ukraine:** Ukraine is a popular destination for surrogacy due to its lower costs. It has laws supporting commercial surrogacy, but it is only available to married heterosexual couples. While the legal framework is somewhat established, recent political instability and conflicts have added risks, and international intended parents may face sudden legal changes or disruptions. For instance, in 2018, several international intended parents faced difficulties in Ukraine when sudden changes in legal procedures caused delays in bringing their newborns home. Understanding these potential pitfalls ahead of time is crucial.
- **Georgia:** Georgia also offers lower-cost surrogacy services. It has a legal framework that supports

heterosexual married couples, but the laws are not as comprehensive as those in the US, which can lead to uncertainties. Additionally, the lack of established guidelines for disputes means potential legal risks for international intended parents.

- **Mexico:** Surrogacy in Mexico can be much cheaper, with some states having surrogacy-friendly laws. However, the legal environment varies significantly between states, and recent regulatory changes have led to confusion and inconsistency. International parents may face challenges in securing legal recognition for their children, making the process more complex than initially expected.

3.5 Countries with Changing or Uncertain Legal Frameworks

In some countries, legal frameworks for surrogacy have changed rapidly, creating uncertainty for intended parents. Countries like **India** and **Thailand** once had established surrogacy programs but in recent years have imposed bans on international surrogacy. Similarly, **Colombia** has seen a rise in surrogacy interest, but legal ambiguities mean intended parents should proceed with caution. When considering surrogacy in countries with less stable legal frameworks, it is vital to do thorough research and understand the potential risks.

Conclusion

When it comes to surrogacy, thorough research and a cautious approach are essential. Before committing to any program, take the time to understand the legal landscape, medical standards, and ethical implications. The United States may come with higher upfront costs, but the peace of mind it offers can save significant emotional and financial strain in the long run.

Chapter 4
Breaking the Silence: How to Address Taboos Surrounding Surrogacy

Surrogacy is a journey filled with hope, love, and the promise of building a family. But despite its growing acceptance, it remains clouded by misconceptions, stigma, and unspoken taboos. These barriers can make an already complex journey even more challenging for intended parents. In this chapter, we will address the common misconceptions and stigmas surrounding surrogacy and touch on why discussing the financial aspects of surrogacy is essential, even though it may feel uncomfortable.

4.1 Common Misconceptions, Stigmas, and Media Portrayals

Despite growing acceptance, there are still numerous misconceptions about surrogacy that can lead to misunderstandings, stigma, or even discrimination. Here are some of the most prevalent:

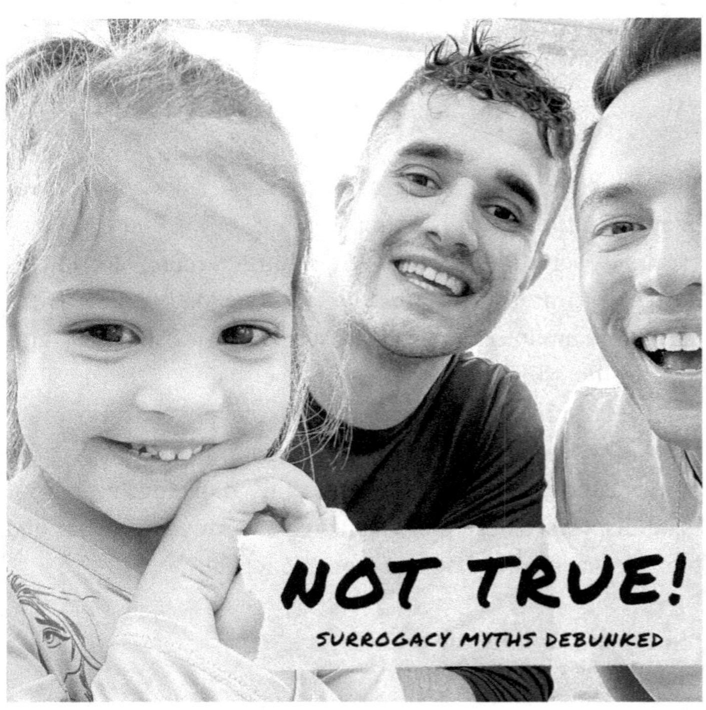

"Why don't you just adopt?"

This is a question many intended parents face, and it's an unfair one. First, anyone familiar with the adoption process will know that it can involve numerous ethical challenges in itself, and, in fact, unethical practices are often more prevalent in adoption than in surrogacy. Adoption is also an intrusive process that can take years to complete, with many unknown outcomes, including the possibility that the adoption may not be finalized. Moreover, it's unfair to assume that people who cannot have children naturally are limited to only one option. Every family-building journey is unique, and intended parents should be free to choose the path that feels right for them without facing judgment or scrutiny.

"What if she keeps the baby?"

This concern is one of the most common fears about surrogacy, but in reality, it is extremely rare. In the United States, especially in states that issue pre-birth orders, the law is designed to protect the rights of the intended parents (IPs). The basic premise is that the surrogate has all the rights during the pregnancy, but once the baby is born, legal parentage shifts to the intended parents. In pre-birth order states, the IPs are recognized as the child's legal parents the moment the baby is born, significantly reducing the risk of legal disputes. These protections make surrogacy a safer and more secure option than many people realize.

"Surrogacy is only for the wealthy."

One of the most pervasive misconceptions is that surrogacy is only an option for the very wealthy. While it is true that surrogacy can be expensive, this perception can overshadow the realities of who turns to surrogacy and why. Surrogacy is often pursued by those who cannot conceive children naturally, including heterosexual couples struggling with infertility, same-sex couples, and single parents. Many intended parents make significant financial sacrifices, save for years, or seek financial assistance to afford surrogacy. The misconception that surrogacy is purely a "luxury" can minimize the very real and emotional desire of individuals and couples to have children.

Media Portrayal and Politicization

Surrogacy is highly politicized in many countries, and with this politicization comes stigma. Many people do not have personal experience with surrogacy, so their understanding is often shaped by how it is portrayed in the media. Unfortunately, stories that aim to shock or scandalize tend to dominate, overshadowing the many successful and ethical arrangements where families are formed in a positive and supportive environment. Balanced and accurate narratives are essential to counteract these misconceptions and reduce stigma.

4.2 Addressing the Taboo Around Finances

Talking about finances can be uncomfortable, especially when it comes to having a child. In many cultures, discussing money in relation to building a family is seen as taboo, making it difficult for intended parents to be open about the realities of the costs involved in surrogacy. However, it is essential to break this silence:

Getting Comfortable with Financial Discussions

For intended parents, becoming comfortable discussing finances is crucial. Surrogacy is a significant investment, and understanding the costs, creating a budget, and planning for contingencies are key to ensuring a smooth journey. Being honest and open about financial expectations can help intended parents navigate this path with more confidence and less stress.

The Importance of Transparency

One of the challenges with surrogacy is the wide range of costs and the lack of transparency in some markets. Having open conversations about what intended parents can expect to spend, and how those costs are broken down, helps demystify the process and provides clarity. This transparency can also reduce the stigma around the cost of surrogacy, making it easier for others to understand the realities that intended parents face.

Practical tips for fostering transparency include asking for detailed cost breakdowns from clinics, agencies, and legal teams, and setting clear financial expectations from the beginning. This helps avoid surprises and ensures a smoother financial journey.

Conclusion

Surrogacy is a life-changing journey, but it is not without its challenges. Misconceptions, stigmas, and the taboo around finances can make the path to parenthood through surrogacy feel daunting. However, by addressing these taboos and openly discussing the realities, we can create a more informed, supportive, and empathetic environment for intended parents and surrogates alike. By sharing our experiences, being transparent about the process, and challenging misconceptions, we can create a more inclusive and empathetic world for all families. Together, we can break the silence and celebrate the joy that surrogacy brings.

In the following chapters, we will dive deeper into the financial aspects of surrogacy, exploring the breakdown of costs, strategies for saving money, and how to plan financially for this journey.

Chapter 5
Creating Your Financial Blueprint: Understanding Surrogacy Costs in the US

Embarking on a surrogacy journey is a significant financial commitment, and one of the biggest concerns for intended parents (IPs) is understanding the costs involved. The purpose of this chapter is to provide a high-level blueprint of the typical expenses associated with surrogacy in the United States, giving IPs a clear overview of what to expect. While the cost can range widely, from around $100,000 to as high as $250,000 or more, this chapter will explain the key elements that drive these costs. In the chapters that follow, we will explore how these costs can be managed, negotiated, and reduced. Although it's impossible to pinpoint an exact figure for every journey, this blueprint will help IPs start planning and prioritizing what's important for them.

5.1 Why Surrogacy in the US Can Be Expensive

The United States is often regarded as the gold standard for surrogacy, and this reputation is built on several factors that contribute to the overall cost. While the benefits of surrogacy in the US—such as robust legal frameworks, high-quality medical care, and comprehensive ethical practices—are invaluable, they also come with a higher price tag. Here's why:

- **Legal Security and Protection:** The US has strong legal frameworks in many states that protect the rights of both intended parents and surrogates. This legal clarity ensures that all parties are aware of their rights and responsibilities, providing peace of mind that is often unmatched in other parts of the world. However, the legal processes, including drafting contracts, securing pre-birth orders, and navigating parental recognition, add to the overall expense. Additionally, international IPs may need legal counsel in their home country to ensure that parentage is legally recognized once they return, which can further add to the cost.

- **High Standards of Medical Care:** The US is home to some of the world's leading fertility clinics, offering state-of-the-art technology and high success rates for IVF procedures. The quality of care, including advanced techniques, personalized treatment plans, and cutting-edge facilities, contributes to the expense but increases the likelihood of a successful pregnancy. This high standard of care also extends to prenatal and delivery care, ensuring the well-being of both the surrogate and the baby.

- **Ethical Practices and Comprehensive Support:** Ethical surrogacy in the US involves thorough screening, fair compensation, legal counsel, and continuous support for surrogates. These practices ensure that surrogates are cared for throughout the process, creating a safer and more ethical environment for everyone involved. However, the high level of care and support provided throughout the journey increases the cost.

5.2 Breakdown of Typical Surrogacy Costs

To better understand where your money will go, let's break down the typical costs associated with a surrogacy journey in the US:

- **Agency Fees:** These can range from $20,000 to $50,000. Agencies coordinate many aspects of the journey, including matching you with a surrogate, coordinating legal and medical appointments, and providing ongoing support.
- **Medical and Fertility Clinic Fees:** Expect to spend between $30,000 to $70,000. This includes IVF treatments, embryo transfers, and other necessary medical procedures.
- **Surrogate Compensation:** Surrogates are typically compensated for their time, effort, and the physical demands of pregnancy. Compensation packages can range from $35,000 to $55,000, with additional payments for specific circumstances (like carrying multiples or undergoing a C-section).
- **Legal Fees:** You will need to budget around $10,000 to $20,000 for legal expenses, which include drafting contracts, securing pre-birth orders, and navigating any other legal requirements specific to your case.
- **Insurance:** Depending on your surrogate's current insurance and the need for additional coverage, insurance costs can vary. For many international IPs,

there's also the expense of newborn insurance, which may cost around $15,000. Ensure that your policies cover all necessary medical care.

- **Miscellaneous Costs:** Be prepared for an additional $5,000 to $10,000 for travel expenses, psychological support, embryo storage, and any unforeseen expenses that may arise during the process.

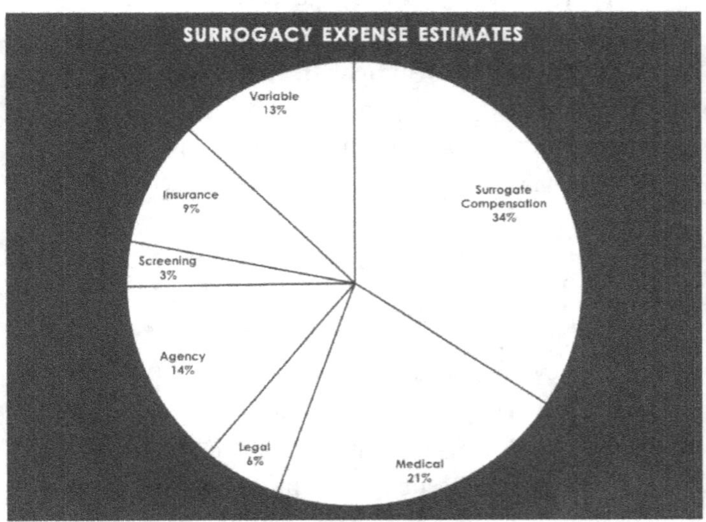

5.3 Budgeting for Surrogacy: Planning and Contingency Funds

Planning for surrogacy requires careful budgeting. Here are some tips to help IPs manage their finances:

- **Create a Detailed Budget:** Start by listing all the expected expenses, including agency fees, medical costs, and legal services. Factor in travel, insurance, and any potential extras that might arise. Having a clear picture of your financial commitments will help you prepare for the journey.

- **Plan for Contingency:** Surrogacy can be unpredictable, and even the best-laid plans can face setbacks. Whether it's a need for additional IVF cycles, unexpected medical expenses, or finding a new surrogate, it's wise to set aside a contingency fund (10-15% of your total budget) to cover any unexpected costs.
- **Understand Payment Schedules:** Surrogacy payments are typically spread out over several months. Understanding when and how payments are due will help you plan your cash flow effectively.

Conclusion

The cost of surrogacy in the US can be overwhelming, with a typical journey ranging anywhere from $100,000 to $250,000 or more. This chapter has provided a high-level blueprint of where those expenses come from, including medical, legal, and surrogate compensation costs. In the following chapters, we will drill down into how these costs can be managed and reduced. While it's difficult to provide a precise number, this financial blueprint helps IPs start making informed decisions, prioritize what's important to them, and budget effectively for their surrogacy journey.

Chapter 6
Cost-Saving Strategies: How to Make Surrogacy More Affordable

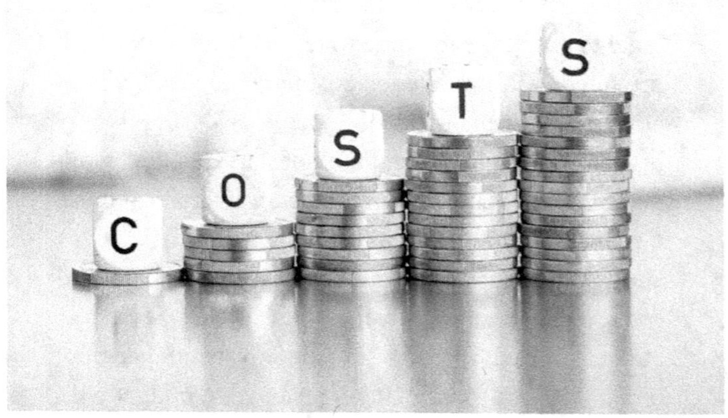

The cost of surrogacy in the United States can be daunting, often ranging from $100,000 to $250,000 or more. However, there are strategies that intended parents (IPs) can use to make the journey more affordable without compromising on quality or safety. This chapter provides practical tips to help reduce costs, identify potential savings, and ensure that IPs can navigate the surrogacy process within their budget. Ultimately, it's essential to decide what's right for you—surrogacy can involve calculated risks, and there are areas where you can cut costs while still adhering to basic surrogacy guidelines.

6.1 Plan and Budget Carefully

Effective cost-saving starts with careful planning and budgeting. The more informed and prepared you are, the easier it will be to avoid unnecessary expenses. Here's how to get started:

- **Research and Compare Providers**: Costs can vary significantly between different agencies, clinics, and legal teams. Take the time to research multiple providers, ask for detailed cost breakdowns, and compare what is included. Sometimes, a slightly higher upfront cost might include services that would otherwise add up, resulting in better overall savings.
- **Create a Detailed Budget**: Break down all anticipated expenses, including agency fees, medical costs, legal services, travel, and insurance. Set a budget for each category and plan for contingencies (about 10-15% extra). Having a detailed budget will help you track spending and avoid going overboard.

6.2 Choosing the Right Fertility Clinic

Selecting a fertility clinic is one of the most important decisions in your surrogacy journey, and it can also be a significant area for cost savings. Since the clinic represents a large percentage of overall costs, it's crucial to find one that is reputable, has great success rates, and offers packages where all costs are known. Here are a few strategies to consider:

- **Look for Clinics in More Affordable States**: The cost of medical care can vary greatly across the United States. Choosing a clinic in a state where the cost of living is lower can help reduce your overall expenses. Additionally, some states have lower IVF and treatment costs, which can make a big difference, especially if multiple cycles are needed.
- **Opt for Clinics with In-House Egg Donor Programs**: If you require an egg donor, consider working with a clinic that has its own egg donor program. Clinics with in-house donors can streamline the process, and their packages are often more affordable than using an external agency. This option could save you at least $10,000 in agency fees.
- **Seek All-Inclusive Packages**: Some clinics offer packages that include multiple services, such as unlimited embryo transfers, medications, and other fertility treatments. These "all-inclusive" or "guarantee" packages can provide peace of mind by setting a fixed price for the IVF process, minimizing unexpected costs. While these packages may seem more expensive upfront, they can save money in the long run, particularly if multiple IVF cycles are needed.
- **Ask Questions and Dig Into Costs**: Make sure to have a detailed discussion with your clinic about their cost structure. Ask whether they offer egg

donor programs, what is included in their packages, and if there are hidden fees. Knowing all costs upfront will help you avoid surprises later.

- **Negotiating with Clinics**: It's okay to negotiate, especially when discussing worst-case scenarios. Make sure to address what will happen if things don't go as planned, and have these details in writing. For example:
  - What happens if fewer eggs are retrieved than anticipated?
  - What if the quality of embryos is lower, requiring another cycle?
  - Are there additional costs for embryo freezing and storage if the process takes longer than expected?

6.3 Decide if You Are Open to an Independent Journey or Agency

Choosing between an independent surrogacy journey and working with an agency is a critical decision that affects both your budget and experience. Here are some insights to help you decide:

- **Independent Journey Considerations**: I am not a huge fan of recommending an independent journey, primarily because surrogates who choose this path may not meet the strict guidelines that agencies enforce. For example, they might have a higher BMI, be a few years older, or have a bad credit history. This, however, does not mean they are incapable of delivering a healthy baby. Reputable clinics will not move forward with a surrogate who is not medically fit, ensuring that no corners are cut.

- ○ **The Pros**: Choosing an independent journey can save on agency fees, but it comes with more legwork. You will still need to arrange for proper medical and psychological screening, background checks, and other steps that agencies typically handle. There are also social media groups, apps, and platforms where you can connect with potential surrogates.
- ○ **The Cons**: One challenge with an independent journey is the lack of a "bridge of communication." It can be uncomfortable discussing finances and personal matters directly with the surrogate without the buffer that agencies provide. Agencies act as intermediaries, managing delicate topics and helping navigate the relationship, which can make the journey smoother for everyone.
- **Working with an Agency**: If you decide to use an agency, I highly recommend looking into smaller, boutique agencies. These often provide a more personalized service, and their fees are generally lower than larger, full-service agencies. As always, do your research, read reviews, and ensure that any agency you consider has a solid reputation and positive feedback.
  - ○ **Negotiating with Agencies**: One of the key areas to address is the matching fee. Ask what happens if you are matched with a surrogate and things don't work out—do you have to pay a whole new matching fee for a second attempt? Additionally,

try to find an agency that does not charge fees until you are matched with a surrogate.

6.4 Consider a First-Time Surrogate

One way to reduce costs is to consider working with a first-time surrogate. Compensation structures are based on experience, and a first-time surrogate will typically cost at least $15,000 less than someone who has done it before. Here are some points to think about:

- **The Cost Difference**: Compensation for first-time surrogates is lower because they haven't yet proven their ability to successfully complete a surrogacy journey. However, this does not mean they are unqualified—almost all surrogates have had their own children, which confirms their ability to carry a pregnancy.
- **Keeping an Open Mind**: While it might feel more reassuring to work with a surrogate who has done it before, first-time surrogates are often very enthusiastic and dedicated. Their excitement about embarking on this meaningful journey can make the experience just as fulfilling, if not more so.

6.5 Optimize the Use of Insurance

Insurance can be one of the largest expenses in a surrogacy journey, but there are ways to optimize and potentially reduce costs:

- **Understand Surrogate's Existing Insurance**: Start by having a professional assess the surrogate's current health insurance policy. Some policies may be "surrogacy-friendly" and cover aspects of the pregnancy, while others may have exclusions. Understanding this early on can prevent unexpected expenses later.

- **Newborn Insurance for International IPs**: I am not an insurance expert and cannot give insurance advice, but I can share some insights. Newborn insurance policies for international IPs are often astronomically expensive, largely due to fear of the high cost of NICUs in the US. However, there are more affordable ACA policies that can be purchased for the baby alone, sometimes for just a few hundred dollars compared to thousands.

  - **Consult a Licensed Local ACA Broker**: It's important to speak with licensed brokers who are not directly tied to surrogacy-specific insurance. Explain your situation honestly and explore options that might allow you to use a temporary US address (like an Airbnb or hotel) for coverage. Remember, your child is considered American from the moment they are born, which opens up different insurance possibilities. Consult experts to find the best and most affordable solution.

6.6 Be Smart About IVF and Medical Costs

Medical costs, particularly those related to IVF, are a significant part of surrogacy expenses. There are several strategies you can use to manage these costs effectively:

- **Choose a Clinic with High Success Rates**: Clinics with higher success rates may seem more expensive, but they can save you money in the long run by reducing the need for multiple IVF cycles. Fewer cycles mean fewer medications, lower lab fees, and reduced overall costs.
- **Use Frozen Embryos**: If you have multiple embryos from a single IVF cycle, consider using frozen embryos for future attempts rather than undergoing a new cycle. This can be much more cost-effective.
- **Medication Savings**: Fertility medications are expensive, but there are ways to reduce costs. Compare prices between pharmacies, and look for online options that may offer discounts. Some fertility clinics have partnerships with specific pharmacies that provide better rates for their patients. You might also consider using generic medications where possible. Additionally, some clinics offer packages where medications are included, potentially reducing the total cost.

6.7 Consider Surrogates From More Affordable States

Surrogacy costs can vary significantly depending on the state where the surrogate lives. Choosing a surrogate from a state with a lower cost of living can lead to savings on compensation, travel, and other expenses. However, ensure that the state's surrogacy laws are favorable to your situation. Here are a few considerations:

- **Check State Laws**: Make sure the state has clear,

supportive surrogacy laws that protect the rights of intended parents.

- **Match with a Surrogate Close to Your Clinic**: Whenever possible, try to find a surrogate who lives in the same state as your fertility clinic. This can save significantly on travel expenses and eliminate the need for a separate "monitoring clinic" near the surrogate's home. If the surrogate lives far from the clinic, you'll need to pay for monitoring services (ultrasounds, bloodwork, etc.) at a clinic that is local to them, as well as travel expenses for major procedures like embryo transfer.
- **Factor in Travel and Monitoring Clinic Costs**: Even if the surrogate lives in a more affordable state, calculate the cost of traveling for medical appointments, legal proceedings, and the birth. Sometimes, savings in compensation are offset by travel expenses, so choosing a nearby surrogate can help streamline these costs.

6.8 Manage Legal and Administrative Costs

Legal fees are essential to a surrogacy journey, but there are ways to keep them under control:

- **Compare Attorneys**: Find surrogacy attorneys who have experience but offer competitive rates. Ask for referrals, read reviews, and interview multiple attorneys to ensure you get the best service for your budget.
- **Clarify Legal Costs Upfront**: Make sure you understand what is included in the attorney's fees and what may be considered extra. Some attorneys

offer flat-fee packages that cover all legal aspects, which can help with budgeting.

- **Negotiating with Lawyers**: One important consideration is what happens if your match with a surrogate breaks, and you need a new contract with a different surrogate. Ask your lawyer if there will be additional fees for drafting a new contract, and ensure you understand how this could affect your budget.

6.9 Explore Financial Assistance Options

Surrogacy is an incredibly expensive undertaking that, unfortunately, is not available to most people. I want to emphasize that I'm not here to create financial hardships for you. If, due to the heavy costs involved, you are considering surrogacy outside of the US, then please try to raise the extra money required to undertake it in the US, if only for the better legal security and peace of mind. Here are some options for managing the financial aspect of surrogacy:

- **Family**: If you have family that is able to help, don't let pride get in the way. If there was ever a time to ask for family assistance, this would be it. Be humble and understand that it's okay to ask for help.
- **Surrogacy Loans**: Some financial institutions offer loans specifically designed for fertility treatments and surrogacy. Interest rates and terms vary, so shop around to find the best deal.
- **Grants and Scholarships**: Some organizations provide grants or scholarships to help with surrogacy and fertility treatment costs. These can be

competitive, but it's worth applying if you meet the criteria.

- **Crowdfunding**: While not for everyone, crowdfunding can be a way to raise money for surrogacy expenses. Platforms like GoFundMe allow friends, family, and even strangers to contribute towards your journey.
- **Payment Over the Journey**: The average surrogacy journey takes anywhere from 16 months to 2.5 years. The journey's entire cost is not paid all at once; it is phased and moves in stages. Use this to your advantage and balance smart financial planning with easing financial anxiety.

6.10 Plan Your Journey Strategically

One of the best ways to manage costs is to plan your surrogacy journey strategically. Consider the following tips:

- **Timing**: Consider the timing of your surrogacy journey. Medical costs and legal services may fluctuate, and certain times of the year may have discounts.
- **Book Travel in Advance**: If you know when you'll need to travel for medical appointments or the birth, book flights and accommodations well in advance to get better rates.
- **Be Prepared for Unexpected Costs**: Even with the best planning, unexpected costs can arise. Setting aside a contingency fund can save you from financial stress if surprises do occur.

Conclusion

Surrogacy in the US can be expensive, but with careful planning and smart strategies, it is possible to make the process more affordable. By understanding where costs come from and how to manage them, intended parents can navigate their surrogacy journey without unnecessary financial strain. In the next chapters, we'll continue to explore how to prioritize expenses, distinguish between essential and optional services, and make informed decisions that best suit your needs and budget.

Chapter 7
Managing Challenges: How to Handle Worst-Case Scenarios in Surrogacy

Embarking on a surrogacy journey is a hopeful and exciting process, but it's also a complex one. While most journeys go smoothly, there are potential challenges and worst-case scenarios that, though rare, can occur. Some situations are unlikely, while others may happen more frequently. Preparing for these situations, knowing how to handle them, and mitigating risks can help ease your mind and give you a sense of control over the journey.

What we found most useful was negotiating terms for worst-case scenarios—many of which probably won't happen—but doing so can provide peace of mind. In this chapter, we'll address some potential issues and offer strategies to navigate them effectively. We'll also introduce the concept of "putting stress in buckets," focusing on what you can control and how to manage the rest.

7.1 Potential Worst-Case Scenarios

Here are some possible scenarios that intended parents (IPs) might face, along with suggestions on how to address them:

- **Failed Embryo Transfers**: Unfortunately, not every embryo transfer leads to a pregnancy. Even with the best medical support, success isn't guaranteed, and multiple attempts may be needed. Over the course of three transfers, it is very likely that at least one will result in a successful pregnancy. However, in the rare case that all three attempts fail, it's almost always recommended to change surrogates. This can cause significant stress, add time, and increase costs, but such situations are rare. After one or two failed transfers, clinics may use alternative fertility methods to increase the chances of a successful pregnancy.
  - **Preparation**: Understand success rates and what factors can affect them. Speak with your clinic about the possibility of multiple transfers and plan your budget accordingly. This way, you'll

be financially and emotionally prepared if the first transfer doesn't succeed.

- o **Mitigation**: Discuss with your clinic the best ways to improve your chances, such as selecting higher-quality embryos, considering pre-implantation genetic testing, or ensuring the surrogate is in the best possible health for transfer. Also, negotiate with your clinic beforehand about what the costs would be if you need to repeat the process. Similarly, ask your agency about their policy if you need to rematch through no fault of your own. Some agencies offer negotiated rematch fees or packages that include unlimited matches. Addressing these concerns upfront can provide peace of mind.

- **Not Getting as Many Donor Eggs or Embryos as Anticipated**: One of the potential challenges is not retrieving as many eggs from a donor as initially hoped, leading to fewer embryos. This can be stressful, especially if you're relying on a specific number of embryos for multiple transfer attempts.

- o **Preparation**: When working with a clinic, ask what happens if fewer eggs or embryos are produced than expected. Ensure you have a plan in place, including potential costs for additional egg retrievals if needed.

- o **Mitigation**: Clinics may have strategies to improve the chances of successful egg retrieval, including optimizing the donor's health and the timing of the retrieval process. Discuss these methods with your clinic and consider negotiating for coverage in case additional cycles are required.

- **Miscarriages and Stillbirths**: Miscarriages, particularly in the first trimester, are not common but can happen. It's a reality that can be difficult to face, but it's essential to be prepared both emotionally and financially. Late-term stillbirths, although rare, can also occur and are just as likely to happen in a surrogacy pregnancy as in a traditional one.
  - **Preparation**: Understand that while miscarriage is a possibility, the odds are generally in your favor, especially with high-quality embryos and a healthy surrogate. Be prepared for the emotional impact and consider counseling support if needed. Financially, you may need to plan for additional transfers if an early miscarriage occurs.
  - **Mitigation**: If a miscarriage happens, allow yourself time to grieve and process the loss. Your clinic can guide you through the next steps, and you may decide to try again when you're ready. As for stillbirths, it's important to remember that while no surrogacy program can "guarantee" a baby, the proper precautions and medical protocols significantly increase the chances of a successful outcome. This is why surrogacy in the US, as discussed in earlier chapters, is seen as a gold standard—thorough screening, quality healthcare, and legal clarity all make the odds favorable. However, understanding that no process is entirely without risk is crucial to maintaining realistic expectations.
- **Medical Complications During Pregnancy**: Pregnancy always carries risks, and surrogacy is no exception. Complications can range from minor

issues that cause anxiety but aren't serious, to more critical situations that require immediate attention.

- **Preparation**: Trust that the surrogate knows her body and will seek help or medical attention if necessary. Make sure you understand your insurance deductibles and maximum out-of-pocket expenses, and familiarize yourself with concepts like "in-network" and "out-of-network" coverage.
- **Mitigation**: Ensure the surrogate has comprehensive health coverage and that additional insurance is arranged if needed. Understanding the policy's coverage limits and network options will help you plan financially and ensure that you're prepared for unexpected medical costs.

- **Legal Challenges or Parental Rights Issues**: Even within the US, legal complications can arise depending on the state where your surrogate resides. Each state has its own set of surrogacy laws, and it's crucial to understand these laws to avoid any surprises regarding parental rights. While rare, issues may emerge if the legal framework is not fully understood or if the necessary documentation is not in place.

  - **Preparation**: Work with experienced legal professionals who specialize in surrogacy law and understand the specific laws of the state where your surrogate lives. Make sure all legal contracts are thorough and in compliance with local regulations. The legal team should ensure that a pre-birth order or other necessary legal steps are completed well before the birth, securing your parental rights. For international IPs, it's crucial to understand the path to parental recognition in your home country. Ensure you know what documents are needed and what the process will be before bringing your baby home. Waiting until you're back home can lead to bureaucratic and legal challenges.

- o **Mitigation**: Stay informed and proactive. Ask your legal team to walk you through the process step by step, ensuring there are no gaps in the legal framework. Being well-prepared and having the correct legal documents in place before the birth will minimize the risk of complications.

- **Surrogate Backs Out of the Agreement**: Until the surrogate is pregnant, she has the right to step back from the contract at any time. While this is uncommon, life can be unpredictable, and situations may arise where a surrogate decides not to proceed. This could be due to personal reasons, such as unexpected family issues, health concerns, or changes in her circumstances.

- o **Preparation**: Ensure the surrogate is fully aware of the commitment involved and has undergone thorough psychological screening to assess her readiness. Solid legal contracts will set clear expectations, but building open and honest communication from the beginning can help prevent misunderstandings.

- o **Mitigation**: Understand that, in practice, the contract becomes enforceable in a meaningful way once the surrogate is pregnant. By this point, surrogates are typically deeply committed to the process. However, if she decides to step back before pregnancy, most agencies have procedures in place to help you find a new match without significant delays. Discuss rematch policies and any associated costs with your agency upfront, so you are prepared if this situation arises.

- **Relationship with the Surrogate Isn't Going Well**: Sometimes, the relationship between IPs and the surrogate doesn't live up to expectations. While this can be tough, it's important to remember that once the surrogate is pregnant, everyone is committed to seeing the journey through. Often, tensions can arise from external factors like hormones, stress, or life challenges the surrogate is facing.
  - **Preparation**: Set realistic expectations and understand that there may be ups and downs throughout the process. Discuss beforehand how you plan to handle potential conflicts or misunderstandings.
  - **Mitigation**: Communication is key. If issues arise, try to address them directly but respectfully. Keep in mind that surrogates have their own lives, and sometimes external stressors might impact their mood or behavior. Also, consider how your actions might affect the surrogate—being overly controlling can push her away. This is where having an agency can be extremely helpful, especially when it comes to sensitive issues like financial arrangements.

7.2 Strategies for Mitigating Risk

While it's impossible to eliminate risk altogether, there are several strategies you can use to mitigate potential issues:

- **Thorough Screening and Vetting**: Make sure everyone involved, from your surrogate to the medical team, is properly screened and vetted. The more experienced and professional your team is, the less likely you are to face complications. Use agencies and clinics that have rigorous standards for screening surrogates, donors, and staff.
- **Detailed Contracts**: Your contracts should address every possible scenario, from failed transfers and emergency medical situations, to what happens if you need to match with a new surrogate. The more thorough the contracts, the fewer chances there are for misunderstandings or disputes.
- **Negotiating Worst-Case Scenarios**: While it might feel uncomfortable to think about what could go wrong, negotiating terms for these situations can provide significant peace of mind. Discussing scenarios like rematching or repeat procedures can help you prepare financially and emotionally.

7.3 Putting Stress in "Buckets"

One helpful strategy for managing stress during the surrogacy journey is to "put your stress in buckets." This means organizing your concerns into categories you can manage and focusing on what you can control, while acknowledging that there are things you cannot control. Here's how it works:

- **Bucket 1: Things You Can Control**
- Examples: Choosing the right providers, ensuring all legal documents are in order, maintaining open communication with your team.
- *Strategy*: Focus your energy on these areas, making sure everything is as prepared and clear as possible. If you can take proactive steps, do so.
- **Bucket 2: Things You Can Influence**
- Examples: The surrogate's comfort during pregnancy, how well your embryo transfers go (though success isn't guaranteed).
- *Strategy*: While you can't fully control these, you can support them. For example, ensure the surrogate has everything she needs to be comfortable and healthy, and work closely with your clinic to optimize the chances of success.
- **Bucket 3: Things Out of Your Control**
- Examples: Natural complications during pregnancy, unexpected legal hurdles, the outcome of embryo transfers.
- *Strategy*: Understand that no matter how much you plan, there are things you cannot change. Worrying won't make them go away, so do your best to manage your anxiety by focusing on what you *can* control. Having a strong support system, whether that's friends, family, or mental health professionals, can help you navigate these stressful moments.

7.4 Preparing for the Unexpected

While the likelihood of facing a worst-case scenario is small, it's still a good idea to be prepared. Some practical ways to prepare include:

- **Having a Contingency Fund**: Budgeting for the unexpected ensures that you won't be blindsided by surprise expenses. It's wise to have extra funds set aside for scenarios like additional embryo transfers, travel costs, or emergency medical procedures.
- **Regular Check-Ins with Your Team**: Maintaining regular communication with your agency, legal team, and clinic helps you stay informed and prepared for any changes. Make sure to ask questions and seek clarity whenever you have doubts.
- **Being Emotionally Prepared**: Surrogacy is a rollercoaster of emotions, and sometimes things don't go as planned. Preparing yourself mentally for potential setbacks can make it easier to cope when challenges arise. Consider seeking support from a counselor or joining a support group for IPs.

Conclusion

Surrogacy is a life-changing journey filled with hope and anticipation, but it's important to be prepared for potential challenges. By understanding worst-case scenarios and knowing how to mitigate risks, you can approach the journey with greater confidence. Remember that while you can't control everything, you can plan, communicate, and build a strong support network. By "putting stress in buckets," you can focus your energy on what matters most, and trust that your team of professionals is there to support you through every step.

Chapter 8
Getting Started: How to Prioritize and Plan Your Surrogacy Journey

Embarking on the surrogacy journey is a significant decision that requires careful thought, planning, and preparation. While the process can seem overwhelming at first, breaking it down into manageable steps can help you navigate the complexities and set a clear path forward. In this chapter, we'll cover how to prioritize essential aspects of your journey, distinguish between what's necessary and what's optional, and guide you through the first steps of your surrogacy process.

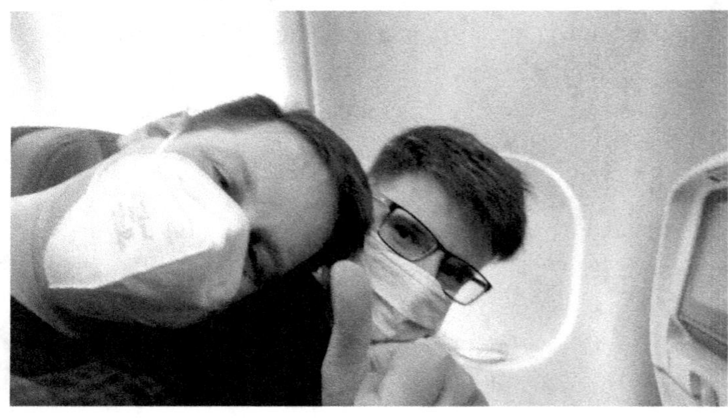

8.1 Understanding the Essentials

Every surrogacy journey is unique, but there are certain essential components that all intended parents (IPs) need to consider. These are the foundational aspects that ensure the process runs smoothly, legally, and ethically. Let's explore what's typically non-negotiable:

- **Legal Contracts and Counsel**: Engaging a knowledgeable surrogacy lawyer is critical. Legal agreements protect the rights of both the IPs and the surrogate, clarifying responsibilities and expectations. Without a solid legal foundation, there can be misunderstandings or even legal disputes, especially if complications arise.
- **Medical Procedures**: Fertility treatments, such as in vitro fertilization (IVF), are at the core of the surrogacy process. Working with a reputable clinic ensures that the surrogate can carry the pregnancy safely and that the embryos are healthy. Proper medical screenings, embryo transfers, and monitoring are all essential steps.
- **Surrogate Compensation and Care**: Ensuring that your surrogate is compensated fairly and receives comprehensive healthcare is a vital part of the surrogacy journey. This includes regular prenatal checkups, emotional support, and covering all pregnancy-related costs. Additionally, it's usually mandatory to buy a life insurance policy for the surrogate, ensuring financial security for her family during the pregnancy.
- **Insurance**: Having the right insurance in place is crucial to avoid unexpected medical expenses. This

includes health insurance for the surrogate and, if you're an international IP, newborn insurance for your child. It's important to have these policies reviewed by an expert to ensure there are no gaps in coverage.

- **Communication and Support Systems**: The surrogacy journey is an emotional one. Having a strong support system, whether that's your partner, family, friends, or a surrogacy coordinator, will make the process less stressful. Clear and honest communication with your surrogate and other involved parties is also essential for a smooth journey.

8.2 Recognizing What's Optional

While there are many essential components, some parts of the surrogacy process are optional and can be customized based on your budget, preferences, and specific needs. Deciding which aspects are optional for your journey can help manage costs effectively:

- **Agency Services**: Some IPs choose to work independently, matching with a surrogate directly and coordinating the journey without the help of an agency. This can save on fees, but requires more legwork. Using an agency can provide peace of mind, as they handle everything from screening to coordination, but it's not strictly necessary if you're comfortable taking on these responsibilities yourself.
- **Egg Donor Agencies**: If you need an egg donor, working with an agency can streamline the process by providing access to pre-screened donors.

However, some clinics have in-house donor programs that are often more affordable. You might also consider looking for egg donors independently through support groups or referrals, though this may require more time and effort.

- **Specialized Insurance Policies**: While certain types of insurance are essential, there are some optional policies (like additional life insurance for the surrogate or supplementary newborn coverage) that may provide extra security but aren't strictly necessary. These should be considered based on your own comfort level and budget.

8.3 Deciding on Matching Points

One of the most important aspects of planning your journey is deciding what's most important to you when matching with a surrogate. These "matching points" are key factors that will shape your experience:

- **Views on Termination**: This is an incredibly difficult topic to think about, but it's essential to address. Some surrogates are not willing to consider termination under any circumstances, while others may have more flexible views. Make sure this topic is discussed early on so that everyone is on the same page.
- **Vaccination Preferences**: Although the COVID-19 pandemic brought vaccination into focus, it's not the only vaccine that might need to be considered. Make sure to discuss vaccination requirements, as these can be a critical matching point between IPs and surrogates.

- **Relationship with the Surrogate**: The relationship between IPs and the surrogate will develop naturally, but it's important to address what type of contact you both want during the journey and after the child is born. Do you want to be involved in every appointment? Would you prefer regular updates or minimal communication? Clarifying this helps manage expectations on both sides.
- **Presence During Delivery**: Discuss whether the surrogate is comfortable with you being present in the delivery room. This can be a significant emotional moment, and setting expectations early ensures there are no surprises on the day of birth.
- **Essential vs. Non-Essential Requirements**: Decide what your absolute must-haves are, but be aware that the more requirements you have, the longer it may take to find a suitable match, and the more expensive the process can become. For example, dietary restrictions are standard (no raw seafood, no deli meats, etc.), but more specific requests, like an organic or plant-based diet, can complicate the process and increase costs. Being flexible where possible can lead to a smoother journey.

8.4 Step-by-Step Guide to Starting Your Surrogacy Journey

Let's walk through the essential steps to get started:

- **Step 1. Consult a Lawyer in Your Home Country (For International IPs):** If you're an international intended parent, the first step is to understand the legal path to parenthood when bringing your baby home. Consulting a lawyer in your home country can help clarify how parental recognition works, ensuring that there are no unexpected legal complications after the birth.

- **Step 2. Choose the Right Clinic:** Your clinic will be a significant part of your journey, so finding one that suits your needs is crucial. Look for clinics that offer comprehensive services, including in-house egg donor programs, all-inclusive packages, and clear cost structures. Reputable clinics will have good success rates and the ability to address all your questions about IVF, embryo transfers, and more.
- **Step 3. Begin the Embryo Creation Process:** Once you've selected your clinic, you can begin creating embryos. For same-sex male couples, this involves several steps:
  - **Sperm Quality Testing**: Testing the sperm quality of one or both partners to determine the best path forward.
  - **Finding an Egg Donor**: If an egg donor is required, this will be coordinated either through the clinic's donor base or an agency.
  - **Starting the IVF Schedule**: Planning and preparing the surrogate and the embryos for transfer.
- **Step 4. Start the Matching Process with a Surrogate:** Finding a surrogate can take time, but it's also possible to match quickly. The process can either be undertaken independently or through an agency, and your match time will depend on your personal requirements and a bit of luck.
  - **Don't Get Discouraged**: Some agencies might tell you there's a long waiting list, but others

might provide a match within a few weeks. Much of this depends on specific requirements and timing. For instance, we found our surrogate within weeks. It just took one call to the agency, which already had a surrogate looking to start her second journey and was a perfect match for us.

- **Important Note**: Once a match is identified, there are still several steps before everything is official. Your surrogate must be medically cleared by your clinic, pass psychological screenings, undergo background checks, and more. This process can take time, so be patient.

- **Step 5. Hire a Lawyer in the Surrogate's State:** Once you have a match, it's crucial to engage a lawyer based in the surrogate's state. Each state has its own surrogacy laws, and a local attorney will understand the ins and outs of the legal landscape, helping to navigate any potential challenges.

- **Step 6. Set Up an Escrow Account:** Always use a third-party escrow company to manage funds. An escrow account ensures that all payments to the surrogate and other involved parties are handled securely and transparently, minimizing the risk of disputes.

- **Step 7. Manage Contracts:** The contract phase can be intense, as it's designed to cover all aspects of the surrogacy journey. Your lawyer will draft the agreements, and you'll have opportunities to ask questions and negotiate terms. We kept things simple by instructing our lawyer to stick to a standard contract format, which worked well for us.

- **Step 8. Finalize Insurance Arrangements:** Determine whether the surrogate has a "surrogacy-friendly" insurance policy. This must be assessed by a specialist who reviews policies for surrogacy. If she doesn't have a suitable policy, you will need to purchase one.

8.5 Navigating the Medical Journey

By now, you have selected an egg donor, created embryos, matched with a surrogate, engaged a lawyer, set up an escrow account, and finalized the contract. Congratulations! Here's what comes next:

- **Preparing for Transfer Day**: The surrogate will undergo several medical preparations before the embryo transfer. There are multiple steps involved to ensure her body is ready, so be patient and keep communication lines open.
- **Transfer Day**: This is a significant milestone, but be prepared for mixed emotions. Successful transfers can happen on the first try, though it's not uncommon for multiple attempts to be needed. Stay optimistic but grounded. We had success on our second try, but I know many who succeeded on the first or third.
- **Pregnancy Tests and Heartbeat Ultrasounds**: After a successful transfer, the first pregnancy test will confirm if the process worked. Celebrate this milestone, but stay cautiously optimistic until you reach the heartbeat ultrasound, usually around weeks 6-7. Reaching this point is a major success, with high chances of a healthy pregnancy following.

8.6 Preparing for the Birth

As the pregnancy progresses, your role will shift:

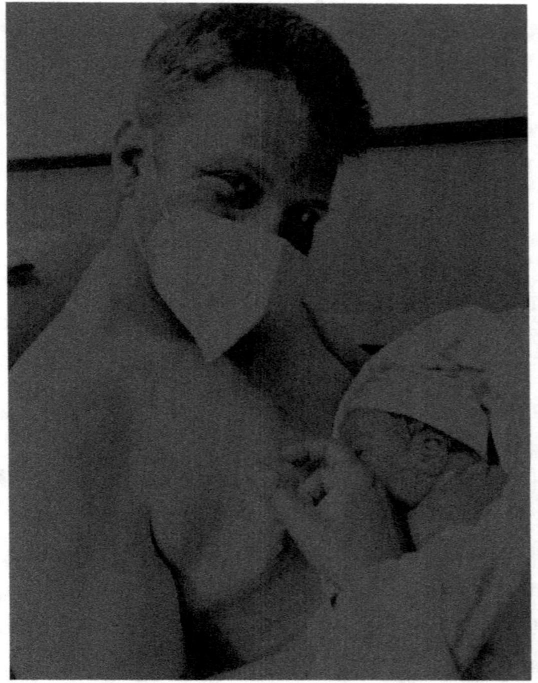

- **The Delivery Experience**: Our own delivery lasted around 36 hours. It's a long and intense process, but if the plan is to be present in the room for delivery, you'll be there when it matters most. Words cannot describe the cathartic moment of seeing your baby's head and cutting the umbilical cord. It's a powerful experience—take it all in.
  - Usually, the baby is placed on the surrogate's chest for a few moments right after birth. If you're uncomfortable with this, it can be

addressed in the pre-birth plan, but in the moment, it may be the last thing on your mind. Within minutes, your baby will be handed to you, and skin-to-skin contact can begin. You'll likely stay in the room with the surrogate for a couple of hours before heading to the maternity ward.

- **Hospital Accommodations**: Most hospitals in surrogacy-friendly states are well-prepared for surrogacy. In most cases, they will do their best to accommodate you by setting up a room for you and your baby while the surrogate has a separate room nearby. Assuming a healthy birth, you'll typically be discharged within 1-2 days.

- **Saying Goodbye to the Surrogate**: Be prepared for a level of emotion you may not have anticipated when it's time to say goodbye to the surrogate. Our personal experience was deeply emotional. After a sleepless night with Noah crying, we went to see our surrogate in the morning. Suddenly, alarms went off, and there was a "code blue." It turned out she had retained placenta, requiring a procedure that led to significant blood loss. It was a terrifying moment, especially after an already emotional week, but thankfully, everything turned out fine.

  - When we said our goodbyes, we couldn't stop crying. There was an overwhelming mix of emotions, and yes, a lingering sense of guilt. It felt unnatural, but I assure you, this does not affect your connection with your baby. The relationship we've maintained with our surrogate remains special to this day.

Conclusion

Starting a surrogacy journey can be both exciting and intimidating, but careful planning and thoughtful prioritization will set you on the right path. By understanding what's essential and what's optional, setting a realistic budget, and taking your first steps with a clear plan, you can approach this journey with confidence. Remember that this is not just a financial or logistical process, but an emotional and life-changing journey. With the right preparation, you can make informed decisions that fit your needs and bring you closer to your goal of starting a family.

In the next chapter, we'll dive deeper into how to build your team of professionals, from agencies to lawyers, to ensure you have the best support every step of the way.

Chapter 9
Building Your Team: How to Choose the Right Providers for Surrogacy

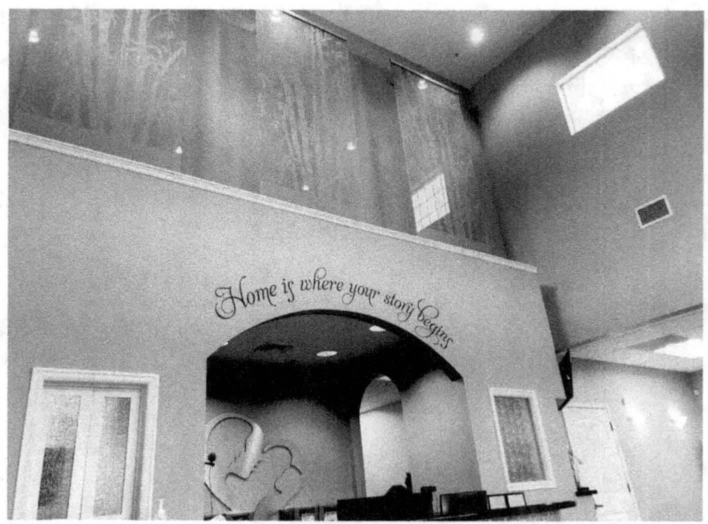

The surrogacy journey is a complex and intricate process that involves many moving parts. One of the most crucial steps is building a strong team of professionals who can guide and support you through each stage. Selecting the right providers—whether it's your agency, legal team, clinic, or other professionals—will play a significant role in ensuring a smooth and successful journey. In this chapter, we will explore how to choose the best professionals and provide tips for evaluating and selecting the right team members.

9.1 Your Surrogacy Team Roadmap

Before we dive into the specifics of each role, it's helpful to have a clear understanding of who will make up your team and at what point during your journey they will be needed. Here's a roadmap of the key professionals involved:

- **Lawyer in Your Home Country (For International IPs)**: If you're an international intended parent, consulting a lawyer in your home country early on is crucial. While there's no need to retain one at the beginning, it's wise to have a consultation to understand how parental recognition will work when bringing your baby home. Have this lawyer on standby to handle any legal steps needed once your journey is complete.
- **Fertility Clinic**: Your clinic will be one of the first professionals you engage, handling everything from fertility treatments to embryo transfers. Choose a reputable clinic that offers comprehensive services and a clear cost structure.
- **Agency (If Not Going Independent)**: If you decide to work with an agency, they will be responsible for matching you with a surrogate and coordinating many aspects of the process. Agencies can handle everything from screening to legal coordination, acting as a bridge between you and the surrogate.

- **Lawyer in the State of Your Surrogate (Once Matched)**: Once you've matched with a surrogate, you'll need a lawyer based in her state to handle all the legal aspects, including contracts and parentage orders. Each state has its own surrogacy laws, so working with someone local ensures you're covered.
- **Third-Party Escrow Company**: To manage payments securely and transparently, a third-party escrow company should be engaged. They will oversee all funds related to the surrogacy journey, including surrogate compensation, medical expenses, and more.
- **Insurance Assessor**: Health insurance is a major aspect of surrogacy, and it's important to have a professional assess the surrogate's insurance policy to determine whether it's "surrogacy-friendly." If not, you'll need to purchase an appropriate policy. International IPs may also need assistance with newborn insurance once the baby is born.

With a roadmap in mind, let's drill down into how to evaluate and select the right professionals for your team.

9.2 Consulting a Lawyer in Your Home Country (For International IPs)

For international intended parents, the journey doesn't end when your child is born. You need to ensure that parental rights are recognized in your home country. Consulting a lawyer early can clarify what steps you'll need to take once your baby is born in the US.

- **Understand Parental Recognition**: Each country has different requirements for recognizing parental rights when a child is born through surrogacy. Know what documents you'll need, whether you'll require a local adoption or legal confirmation, and any other steps you'll be required to follow to bring your baby home.

- **Find a Lawyer with Experience in International Surrogacy**: Look for lawyers who specialize in family law and surrogacy. It may also be helpful if they have experience handling cases involving US-born children, as they'll better understand the documentation needed.

- **Have a Lawyer on Standby**: While you may not need to retain a lawyer until later in your journey, it's helpful to consult one early on and have them ready to step in when the time comes. This ensures a smoother transition once your baby arrives.

9.3 Selecting a Fertility Clinic

Your clinic will be central to the success of your surrogacy journey, as they will handle IVF procedures, embryo transfers, and other essential medical steps. Here's how to choose the right one:

- **Success Rates**: Research the clinic's success rates for IVF, embryo transfers, and working with surrogates. While high success rates are promising, ask for detailed explanations on what those numbers mean. A clinic with good results may be worth a higher price.

- **Location and Accessibility**: If possible, choose a clinic that's close to your surrogate's location. This can save costs related to travel and monitoring appointments. If the surrogate lives far from the clinic, you may need to pay for a monitoring clinic to handle her IVF cycles, ultrasounds, and check-ups.
  - *Tip*: Ensure you understand the cost implications of using a monitoring clinic. While it may be necessary, especially for long-distance arrangements, having the surrogate close to the main clinic can simplify logistics and reduce expenses.
- **Range of Services**: Look for clinics that offer all-inclusive packages, including medications, embryo storage, and coordination with egg donors if needed. Packages can help manage costs more effectively by minimizing unexpected expenses. Also, check if the clinic has an in-house egg donor program, as this can save costs compared to going through a separate agency.
- **Comfort Level and Communication**: Choose a clinic where you feel comfortable and supported. The staff should be responsive, empathetic, and willing to answer all your questions. This is an emotional process, so having a team that communicates clearly and supports you is essential.

9.4 Deciding on an Agency or Going Independent

One of the first decisions you'll make is whether to work with a surrogacy agency or manage the process independently. Each path has its benefits and challenges:

- **Using an Agency**: Agencies can simplify the process by handling everything from surrogate matching to coordinating with medical and legal professionals. They act as a bridge of communication between you and the surrogate, which is especially helpful for sensitive discussions like finances. Agencies also handle complex logistics, saving you time and stress.
  - *Pros*: Convenience, professional guidance, streamlined process, and reduced stress.
  - *Cons*: Higher costs due to agency fees.
  - **Choosing the Right Agency**: Look for agencies with strong reputations, transparency in costs, and services that align with your needs. Consider smaller, boutique agencies if you prefer personalized service and lower fees.
  - **Key Tip**: Discuss rematch policies. Ask what the costs would be if the first match doesn't work out. Some agencies offer packages that include unlimited matches or negotiated rematch fees.
- **Independent Journeys**: Managing an independent journey means finding a surrogate yourself and coordinating all legal, medical, and financial aspects. While it can save money, it also requires more effort.
  - *Pros*: Lower costs, more direct control over the process, and potentially quicker matching.
  - *Cons*: More logistical responsibility, and you must handle screenings, contracts, and coordination on your own.
  - **What to Consider**: If you choose to go independent, ensure the surrogate undergoes the same thorough screening as she would through an agency. Many clinics offer comprehensive

medical and psychological screenings, but you'll still need to do background checks and reference calls. Understand that independent surrogates may not meet agency standards, but that doesn't mean they aren't capable of carrying a healthy pregnancy.

9.5 Hiring a Lawyer in the Surrogate's State

Once matched, having a lawyer based in the surrogate's state is essential. Each state has its own surrogacy laws, so local expertise is crucial.

- **Specialization in Surrogacy Law**: Ensure your attorney specializes in surrogacy. They should be well-versed in drafting contracts, securing parental rights, and understanding the nuances of the state's legal framework.
- **Contracts and Parental Rights**: Your lawyer will draft and review contracts, ensuring they cover everything, including compensation, legal rights, and contingency plans. For international IPs, consult a lawyer in your home country to ensure that the documents align with what's needed for parental recognition back home.
- **Negotiating for Worst-Case Scenarios**: Be proactive in addressing what happens if you need a new contract for a different surrogate, or if other legal challenges arise. This upfront negotiation can save you time and stress later.

9.6 Engaging a Third-Party Escrow Company

An escrow account managed by a third-party company ensures that payments are secure, transparent, and timely.

- **Why Use Third-Party Escrow?**: While some agencies manage funds, it's still advisable to use an independent escrow company. This avoids potential conflicts of interest and ensures that payments, such as surrogate compensation and medical expenses, are handled fairly.
- **Choosing the Right Company**: Look for companies specializing in surrogacy escrow management. They should have clear processes, transparent fees, and excellent communication. Knowing your funds are handled securely can offer peace of mind throughout the journey.

9.7 Working with an Insurance Assessor

Insurance is a critical part of the surrogacy journey, and navigating it can be tricky. An insurance assessor helps you understand your options and ensures you have the right coverage.

- **Assessing Surrogacy Insurance**: Insurance assessors will review the surrogate's current policy to determine if it's "surrogacy-friendly." If it's not, they can help you find an appropriate policy. Be honest about your surrogacy plans when consulting an assessor, as not all policies will cover surrogacy pregnancies.

- **Newborn Insurance for International IPs**: If you're an international intended parent, you'll need to consider newborn insurance. High-priced specialty policies often prey on fear, but there are more affordable ACA policies available. Consult a local ACA broker who understands surrogacy insurance, and be upfront about your situation. This will ensure you find the best option without unnecessary costs.

9.8 Tips for Building Your Team

- **Do Your Research**: Take time to thoroughly research each provider. Look for reviews, testimonials, and ask for recommendations. Understand their strengths, weaknesses, and how they handle challenges. A quick Google search often isn't enough when it comes to surrogacy providers. Many of the most valuable insights come from intended parents (IPs) who share their experiences in social media groups dedicated to surrogacy. Joining as many of these groups as possible can help you uncover the true reputation of a provider—whether it's good, bad, ugly, or indifferent. These communities can provide candid feedback and advice that might not be found through official reviews or company websites.
- **Interview Multiple Providers**: It's okay to interview multiple agencies, clinics, or lawyers before making a decision. Prepare a list of questions and don't hesitate to ask about their experiences,

success rates, and how they handle specific scenarios.

- **Negotiate Terms**: Many services, including clinics, agencies, and legal teams, are open to negotiation. Even if prices can't be lowered, you can often gain clarity on what the services will cover. Ask about rematch policies, costs for additional transfers, and other contingency arrangements.
- **Ensure Compatibility**: Beyond professional qualifications, make sure you feel comfortable with your team. Surrogacy is a long and emotional journey, and you want people who understand your needs, respond to your concerns, and share your values.

Conclusion

Building the right team is one of the most important steps in your surrogacy journey. The right professionals will not only provide expertise but also guide and support you through each stage, making the process smoother and less stressful. Take the time to evaluate and select your team carefully, and don't be afraid to ask questions and seek clarity. By surrounding yourself with the right people, you can embark on your journey with confidence, knowing that you are supported every step of the way.

In the next chapter, we'll discuss setting realistic budgets and how to differentiate between essential and optional components of the surrogacy process to help you plan financially.

Chapter 10
Final Thoughts:
Encouragement and Next Steps
for Intended Parents

Embarking on a surrogacy journey is an emotional, complex, and deeply personal experience. Whether you are just beginning to explore this option or are already well along the way, it's important to remember that the journey to parenthood, while challenging, is also incredibly rewarding. As we reach the end of this guide, I want to offer some final reflections and words of encouragement.

10.1 A Journey Like No Other

Surrogacy is not just a medical or legal process; it's a journey that brings together people from different walks of life, united by the hope of creating a family. Every step—from the initial decision to pursue surrogacy, through the highs and lows of the process, to the moment you hold your child for the first time—carries its own set of emotions and experiences. For many intended parents (IPs), the journey can be overwhelming, but it's also a path that is filled with love, resilience, and joy.

As you navigate this journey, there will be moments of doubt and uncertainty. You might feel overwhelmed by the logistics, financial considerations, or the emotional ups and downs. This is all normal. Remember that you are not alone in this; there are countless other IPs who have walked this path, faced similar challenges, and ultimately found their way to parenthood.

10.2 Encouragement and Support for Intended Parents

Surrogacy is an incredible undertaking, and it requires a lot of courage, patience, and trust. There will be times when it feels like things are out of your control, and that's okay. It's natural to have concerns and fears, but try to focus on the bigger picture—the beautiful life you're working so hard to create.

- **Lean on Your Support System**: You don't have to go through this journey alone. Lean on your partner, family, friends, and professionals. Whether it's sharing your excitement, expressing your fears, or asking for practical help, having a strong support network can make all the difference.
- **Celebrate the Milestones**: Each step forward, no matter how small, is a victory. Whether it's finding the right clinic, signing a contract, matching with a surrogate, or hearing the first heartbeat, take the time to celebrate these milestones. They are all important parts of your journey.
- **Trust the Process and Your Team**: You've carefully selected your team of professionals—your clinic, agency, legal advisors, and others. Trust their expertise, and don't be afraid to ask questions or

seek clarification if there's something you don't understand. They are there to guide you and ensure that your journey goes as smoothly as possible.

10.3 Overcoming the Challenges

Every surrogacy journey is different, and no two experiences are exactly alike. You may face challenges along the way, but these obstacles do not define your journey. Instead, they are part of what makes the process unique. It's important to be prepared, to plan carefully, and to know what to expect, but also to be flexible and adaptable when things don't go exactly as planned.

Remember that setbacks are not failures. Each challenge you overcome brings you one step closer to your goal. Surrogacy is a testament to your love, perseverance, and commitment to building your family, and that strength will carry you through the tough times.

- **Stay Informed, But Don't Overwhelm Yourself**: While it's important to educate yourself about the surrogacy process, try not to get overwhelmed by information overload. Focus on what's most relevant to your journey and rely on your team for guidance.
- **Take Care of Yourself**: The surrogacy process can be physically and emotionally draining. Make sure you're taking care of yourself—both mentally and physically. Practice self-care, and consider seeking professional support if you're struggling with the emotional demands of the journey.

10.4 Reflecting on the Experience

One of the most beautiful aspects of surrogacy is that it brings people together. The relationship you build with your surrogate, the connection you make with your support team, and the community of other IPs you become a part of—these are bonds that can last a lifetime. Many IPs find that the journey, while challenging, also brings unexpected moments of connection, kindness, and understanding.

When you look back on your surrogacy journey, you'll be able to see how far you've come. The fears you had at the beginning, the difficult decisions you had to make, and the uncertainties you faced—they all led to the moment when you held your child in your arms. That moment will make everything worth it, and you will know that every step, every challenge, and every victory was part of a story that led to your family.

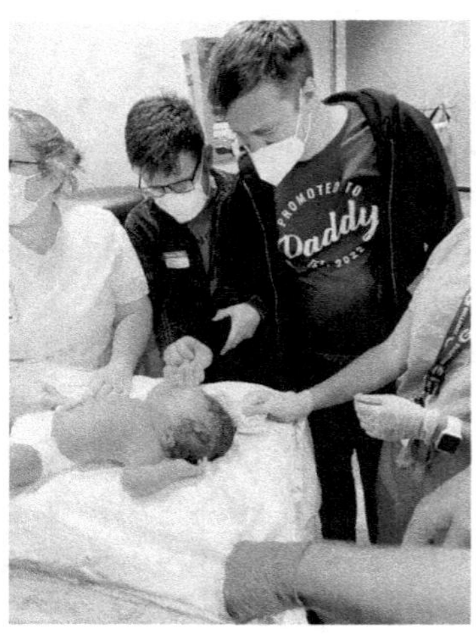

10.5 The Gift of Surrogacy

Surrogacy is a remarkable and beautiful gift—one that brings the joy of parenthood to those who might not otherwise have had the chance. It's a journey that requires patience, trust, and a leap of faith, but it is also filled with hope, love, and new beginnings.

For some IPs, surrogacy is the culmination of years of dreams and planning. For others, it's a new path they never thought they'd walk. Wherever you are on your journey, know that the decision to pursue surrogacy is an act of courage and love. It's a testament to your desire to create a family and to share your life with a child.

10.6 Final Thoughts and Moving Forward

As you move forward with your surrogacy journey, keep these final thoughts in mind:

- **Stay Hopeful**: Even when things get tough, stay hopeful. The road may be long, but the destination is worth every step. Surrogacy is a journey of hope, and that hope will carry you through the challenges.
- **Embrace the Unexpected**: Surrogacy, like life, is unpredictable. Embrace the unexpected moments, and try to find joy even in the uncertainties. The journey may not always go as planned, but it will lead you to where you're meant to be.
- **Focus on What Matters Most**: Throughout the journey, you may encounter many decisions, challenges, and emotions. When it gets overwhelming, come back to what matters most—

your desire to create a family and the love that drives that desire.

I hope this book has provided you with useful insights, practical advice, and the encouragement you need to move forward on your surrogacy journey. Surrogacy is a unique and beautiful way to build a family, and while it may come with its own set of challenges, it's also an experience filled with incredible rewards.

As you take each step forward, know that you are part of a community of intended parents who understand what you're going through. You are not alone, and there are many who are cheering you on, supporting you, and wishing you all the best on this remarkable journey.

* * *

This concludes the surrogacy guide, and I hope it has equipped you with the knowledge, confidence, and support to embark on your surrogacy journey. Remember, you are doing something amazing, and every step you take brings you closer to creating the family you've always dreamed of. Good luck, and may your journey be filled with hope, joy, and love.

Your Next Steps: Stay Connected

Thank you for taking the time to read this book. I hope it has provided you with valuable insights and the confidence to navigate your surrogacy journey. While this book is designed to give you all the essential information, I know that each surrogacy journey is unique and can raise more questions along the way.

1. Connect with Surrogacy Guidance for Additional Support: If you'd like more personalized guidance or have specific questions, you can reach out through Surrogacy Guidance. Our team is here to offer advice and support tailored to your needs. Feel free to book a consultation if you'd like to discuss your unique situation and explore your options further.

2. Stay Updated with News and Tips: Surrogacy is a complex field that can change over time. If you'd like to receive occasional updates, practical tips, and insights, consider subscribing to our newsletter. It's a simple way to stay informed and keep up with the latest developments in the surrogacy world.

3. Join a Community of Intended Parents: Surrogacy can be a deeply personal and emotional journey, but there are many others walking this same path. If you'd like to connect with other intended parents, consider joining our online community. It's a welcoming space where people share experiences, offer support, and celebrate milestones together.

To learn more or explore any of these resources, visit Surrogacy Guidance. Wishing you all the best on your journey to building the family you've dreamed of.

Acknowledgments

I would like to extend my heartfelt gratitude to my life partner, Alex, for his unwavering support and partnership throughout our surrogacy journey and in every aspect of our lives together. Our son, Noah, is the light of our lives and the inspiration behind this book.

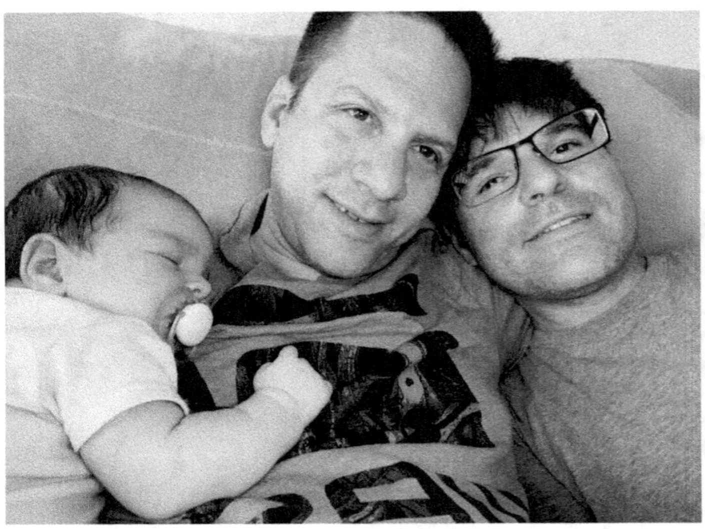

I am also deeply grateful to the professionals who have guided us along the way, providing invaluable insights and support. To the countless intended parents I've worked with, thank you for sharing your stories and experiences, which have greatly enriched this guide.

On a personal note, I want to dedicate this book to my dad, who passed away the week we found out we were "pregnant." His memory inspires me to share this journey with others.

Finally, to all the readers, thank you for taking this journey with me. I hope this book provides you with the knowledge and confidence you need as you navigate your own surrogacy path.